I0440424

Sex Addiction

Get on the Road to Recovery and Learn to Live and Love Life Again

By Jake Roberts

Introduction

I want to thank you and congratulate you for downloading the book, *"Sex Addiction: Get on the Road to Recovery and Learn to Live and Love Life Again"*.

This book contains proven steps and strategies on how to identify and overcome sex addiction.

You will learn about the common symptoms that may be an indication that you are addicted to sex. Check them out to see if you are suffering the symptoms. Learn what causes sex addiction and the effects that it can bring to your life, your partner and your loved ones around you.

In the succeeding chapters, discover steps and strategies to break and overcome sex addiction. Follow the steps and see yourself on the road to recovery. You will also read a chapter on how to avoid relapse while you are on your way to complete freedom. Sex is beautiful and it can be enjoyed to its full passionate potential.

Thanks again for downloading this book, I hope you enjoy it!

Why You Should Read This Book

This book will help you understand that sex addiction is real and that it should be addressed and treated.

You do not have to live a life in the claws of sex addiction forever – you can get out and live free. You can enjoy life, emotional and physical sensations, and shameless intimacy.

This book will help you realize that sex is a gift and you can enjoy it. If you are suffering from sex addiction, then use the strategies that are outlined in this book to help you get started and to stay on the road to recovery.

Remember, there is hope for you!

Copyright

© 2015

All rights reserved. No part of this book may be reproduced or transmitted in any form or by any means, electronic, mechanical, photocopying, recording, or otherwise, without the prior written permission of the publisher.

Disclaimer

The information provided in this book is designed to provide helpful information on the subjects discussed. This book is not meant to be used, nor should it be used, to diagnose or treat any medical condition. For diagnosis or treatment of any medical problem, consult your own physician. The publisher and author are not responsible for any specific health or allergy needs that may require medical supervision and are not liable for any damages or negative consequences from any treatment, action, application or preparation, to any person reading or following the information in this book. Any references included are provided for informational purposes only and do not constitute endorsement of any websites or other sources. Readers should be aware that any websites listed in this book may change.

Table of Contents

Why I wrote this Book

Why You Should Read This Book

Introduction

Chapter 1: Different Types of Sex Addiction

Chapter 2: Symptoms, Causes & Effects of Sex Addiction

Chapter 3: Bust the Myths About Sex Addiction

Chapter 4: Sex Addiction Is A Real Problem

Chapter 5: Break Free From Sex Addiction

Chapter 6: How to Overcome Porn Addiction

Chapter 7: Develop New Behaviors to Prevent Relapse

Chapter 8: A Picture of Recovery from Sex Addition

Bonus Chapter: Recovery for Partners of Sex Addicts

Conclusion

Different Types of Sex Addictions

Sex addiction, also known as sexual dependence, is a compulsive engagement in any sexual activity regardless of the negative consequences that attached to it. Clinically, this term describes someone who is unable to control his sexual urges and behaviors.

There are many types of sex addictions. It is often difficult to identify if someone is struggling with this compulsion.

Following are some information on common types of sex addictions:

- Sex/Love Addiction

  A person with a sex/love addiction may be passionately obsessed with a romantic partner or they easily engage in co-dependent relationships. Pathological behaviors include sexual obsessions, sexual promiscuity, erotomania, nymphomania, hyper-sexuality and paraphilic drives and desires. A person with such mental or neurological disorder can be noticeably impulsive, extremely sexual and seductive.

  However, there are also cases when a person with sex addiction may show signs of emotional or sexual anorexia – this means that the person avoids getting involved in relationships because he fears that he cannot control his emotional and sexual urges.

- Pornography Addiction

  While hyper-sexuality is a common symptom of sexual addiction, experts describe porn addiction as passive, which is why it is harder to diagnose. It is a compulsive behavior that is characterized by frequent use of pornographic material to the extent that it causes grave negative consequences to a person's social, mental, physical, and financial health. Some people use porn to satisfy their sexual urges and obsession. Others use it to add pizzazz to their relationships. The result, however, is quite contrary. Porn actually can make a person less responsive sexually; it prevents people from socializing and having intimacy with their partners. They get pleasure and contentment from viewing naked bodies and watching the act instead of actually enjoying the physical gratification of actual lovemaking. Likewise, a person who has porn addiction may become more demanding or unusually rough because of the influence of his addiction on his mind and emotions. He will most likely spend less time for personal interactions because of excessive time dedicated to viewing pornography.

- Exhibition and Voyeurism

  Exhibitionists expose their private parts – breasts, buttocks or genitals – in public or semi-public environments. The reason behind this behavior could be sexual satisfaction, amusement or to cause shock to other people. Also called indecent exposure, an exhibitionist may actually be seeking attention from others but he has no desire to get involved in a relationship.

  Voyeurism, on the other hand, is the habit of spying on and having sexual interest in people who are engaged in private intimate actions and behaviors. A person with this addiction is obsessed in observing people engaged intimate acts, such as sexual activity or undressing. They will even go so far as secretly take videos or photographs of the activity for his interest. He does not have a desire to have direct interaction with the object of his interest.

Other Types of Sex Addictions

- People who like sex that is based on pain - Pain exchange sex is an activity that associates sexual pleasure with pain
- People who fantasize about sex all the time - Fantasy sex is about an obsession concerning a fantasy sex life that can be so overwhelming it stops a person from having genuinely love in sexual relationships
- People who use sex seductively - Seductive sex involves charming and manipulating others into having numerous sexual relationships
- People who prefer intrusive sex - Intrusive and exploitive sex addicts touch other people in a sexual manner without their permission. This usually happens when one person has significant authority over another.
- People who have various anonymous sex without emotions – In this setting, feelings are aroused by strangers and there is no personal relationship formed
- People who trade sex for money
- People who exploit others for sex

Symptoms, Causes and Effects of Sex Addiction

There are many different factors that can contribute to an addiction to sex. The most common cause is brain stimulation – when someone has been engaged in sex or sex-related activities, his brain may become wired to having a compulsive sexual behavior. Other causes include anxiety, depression and even sexual abuse.

You can identify a person with sex addiction by several indicators in his behavior. Other symptoms can be physical while others can be emotional. The most prevalent physical symptom in people with sex addictions is exhaustion and feeling powerless due to emotional or sexual obsessions. People with sex addiction will not have healthy emotional boundaries. They may fear being abandoned, so they stay in unhealthy relationships or move from one relationship to another. They usually feel incomplete, empty, lonely and guilty so they sexualize their feelings.

The physical effects of sex addiction are severe. Most men and women who have sexual addictions suffer from venereal diseases. Another side effect of this risky, compulsive behavior is unwanted or unplanned pregnancy. Other consequences include: physical exhaustion, financial difficulties, being arrested for inappropriate acts, career loss and even physical injuries.

To get a grip on your behavior and keep yourself from suffering any of the abovementioned consequences, it is best to identify if you are suffering from sex addiction. Assess yourself through the following elements:

- Are you making sexual choices that make your life unmanageable?
- Has sex become a ritual to you?
- Do you promise to change your sexual ways yet fail to do so?
- Do you feel powerless over your emotional behavior towards sex?
- Are you ashamed or embarrassed over your sexual acts?

While it is hard to diagnose this rather destructive, compulsive behavior, checking yourself against the questions will help you get on the road to recovery. The first step is to recognize the problem and your need for change.

Bust the Myths about Sexual Addiction

If you want to break free of sexual addiction, know that the truth will set you free. Some lies and misconceptions have been around so long that people have come to believe them and stopped them from getting out of the pit of sexual addiction.

Media has portrayed sexual addiction as the norm. Even conventional therapists have advised that it is acceptable for open-minded people to indulge in pornography and masturbation. Some cultures even encourage prostitution. The biggest lie that the world shouts: "Do it, as long as it feels good."

In real life, everything may be permissible but not everything is beneficial. It can feel good to masturbate and exhibit in public. It can feel good to look at pictures and videos of naked people and those having sex. It can even feel good to be on drugs or get drunk. It can also feel good to overeat until you become obese. But everything has its consequences; some more terrible than others.

Here are some myths that have kept people from breaking free of their addiction to sex:

Myth : Sex can be a good stress reliever.

Fact: Sex is an intimate and loving bond between your partner and you. It is not a tool to relieve or manage your stress. If used to alleviate stress levels, then it can be abused like food and liquor. Abusive sex degrades and does not enhance intimacy. If you under an enormous amount of stress then you should face it. Manage your time, control your emotions, seek professional help – but never use sex to cope with it.

Myth: Porn isn't a problem because almost everyone uses it.

Fact: Just because everyone else does it, that doesn't mean that it is right. Pornography does not make you more of a man. It does not make you a better lover. It actually destroys the sanctity and beauty of intimacy by making sex as a public viewing material. It has a damaging effect on your mental and emotional health.

Myth: My sex drive is greater than my partner's. He or she is only close-minded or uptight.

Fact: There are two sex drives: a natural loving one and an addictive one. When you think that your drive is greater, you might actually be suffering from a sexual addiction and you are using your partner to satisfy you. Again, sex is a loving, intimate bond meant to give both of you pleasure.

Myth: Masturbation addiction is not real.

Fact: Take anything in moderation – food, drink, exercise, hobbies, and yes, even sex. Any substance or activity used or done in excess can lead to an addiction.

Myth: Addictions are good for you as long as they are positive and make you feel good.

Fact: Positive addiction does not exist. There is no such thing because all forms of addictions are self-destructive.

Myth: There are certain substances are addictive and you cannot prevent that.

Fact: The substance used might be addictive. For example, people can smoke marijuana and not be addicted to it; doctors use morphine in medicinal form during surgeries and people do not get addicted to it; people drink alcohol, but not all of them become alcoholics. Addiction, then, is not about the substance. It lies in a person's choice about using the substance. Sex addiction is a choice.

Myth: An addiction is a failure of morality.

Fact: Addiction and morality are different things. For instance, molesting a child is a moral issue, not an addictive issue. Different kinds of sex addictions can be addictive and still conform to moral standards, but they can be very destructive nonetheless.

Myth: Sex addictions are hereditary.

Fact: It is not in the genes. Many people who have parents who are alcoholics and they do not get addicted to alcohol. Again, sex addiction is a choice that people make to escape the stress of life and cover their weaknesses.

The Biggest Lie: Sexual addiction is normal and acceptable. There is no need to change.

The Biggest Truth: Sexual addiction is a compulsive behavioral problem that can lead to many negative consequences AND you need to change. The good news is that you can escape from this addiction! In the following chapters, you will find out how you can be free and stay free from the bondage of sexual addiction.

Sex Addiction is a Real Problem

Sex addiction is not a myth – it is real and it can cause dire consequences.

Sexual addiction is not only characterized by a strong desire to have sex. It may also be depicted as having an addictive masturbation, a compulsiveness to watch porn or flirt. A person is a sex addict when his behavior towards sex gets out of control and this compulsive behavior begins to have a negative effect on his life.

These compulsive feelings and obsessive behaviors can cause a great deal of hopelessness, confusion and shame for the sex addict. People with sexual addictions are often in a state of denial even if they find their life unmanageable. Sex addiction usually takes up a great deal of energy, and sex addicts find that it causes relationship breakdowns, legal issues, career problems and a degrading loss of interest in things that are non-sexual.

Here are some signs that make it apparent that people have sexual addiction problems.

1. They lead a double life.

   They regularly cheat on their partner. They have a mistress or extra girlfriends. They have a secret sex life. They have a compulsive desire for sexual gain; everything is about them and what they can get.

2. They compromise personal relationships.
   Infidelity is not just about having sex with another person when you are already committed to someone else. It can also mean people viewing sex-related materials and going to sex-related places and events to indulge your compulsive behavior without the knowledge of their partner.

3. They are engage in explicit sexual escapades.
   They do not feel satisfied with sex with one or the same person and they attempt more exciting sexual adventures with other people. They want the high stimulus that these adventures provide. Standard lovemaking becomes a bore for them so they seek sexual variety.

4. They seek out sexually explicit material all the time
   They have such a preoccupation with sex that they constantly seek any sex-related media. It is not about enjoying occasional porn – but consistently

seeking out and enjoying such materials to the extent of being
unproductive at other things.

5. They oft get in trouble with the law.
   Because they engage in many sex-related activities that are mostly illegal –
   like exhibitionism, sex with prostitutes or minors, etc. They get involved in
   offensive activities that bring shame and embarrassment to their partner
   and families.

6. They have negative feelings about their compulsive behavior.
   They like what they do and will do everything to satisfy that desire, but
   they feel guilty, remorseful, shameful and even suicidal. Their life becomes
   unmanageable and yet they may still be in denial. Because they feel
   compelled to do something that is abnormal, they may hate themselves
   and this intense feeling creates a bad behavioral pattern for their life.

While sex addiction may sound like fun, it really isn't. It becomes a destructive
cycle that cannot be stopped unless the addict gets help. It is a behavior, not just
a physical condition. Self-love, self-knowledge and a good approach will help a
sex addict get on the road to recovery. He can get his life back in control.

Break Free from Sex Addiction

People who are suffering from any form of addiction will usually feel that "It is so hard to overcome and I'm stuck with this" or "I can't do it." When they use an ineffective approach, those thoughts may probably be right.

Fortunately, there is an effective approach to breaking free from sex addiction. While you may feel that you are stuck in the mire and mud of this destructive behavior, there is a way out.

Maybe you have tried to change but you have failed. It does not matter. The right approach coupled with proper guidance can help you overcome your addiction. Here are a few important factors that need to be developed if you are to succeed in your endeavor to change and be on the road to recovery.

1. Be honest.

Do not lie to yourself or your partner about your sexual addiction and sexual activities. You may think that being honest can be hard, but you can stop lying. It is a free will choice. No medication or therapy can help you tell the truth – you need to decide to do it. Ask help, if you need, about admitting porn addiction, using prostitutes, addictive masturbation and other sexual activities.

Do not rationalize it with "I'm just having fun. It's harmless." If you want to be free, decide to be honest. This way, your partner and other people around you, such as a life coach or therapist, can help and guide you better.

2. Make the effort by using positive motivation.

Negative discipline never works well. When the approach to dealing with sexual addiction is based on scare and guilt tactics, the methods will absolutely fail. When a person who suffers from sex addiction feels humiliation, he will not want to expose himself to change. He should be supported in a loving and accepting environment where he can be free to admit his weakness and develop strengths to overcome his addiction.

3. Face and do not repress the addictive desires.

Most of conventional therapies advise their patients to stay away from factors that bring on his desires. For example, stop watching movies that might stimulate your sexual desire. Or stay away from magazines and the internet. Or take medication. However, while a person with sexual addiction may try to stay away and repress his desire, it does not address the real issue. The key is to face these desires and overcome them head-on. A good counselor or therapist will help a patient overcome his desires even in stressful and trying situations.

How to Overcome Porn Addiction

Porn addiction is one of the most prevalent sex addictions. It is not easy to identify and people have a hard time admitting and recognizing this addiction. Nevertheless, with enough resolve, one can be free from it.

Following are some strategies on how to overcome porn addiction:

1. Make a decision to stop turning to pornography every time you are in pain or discomfort.

    Remember that stress is a part of life. So are physical pain, frustration, anxiety, embarrassment and depression. And these things are temporary. If you take refuge in port every time you encounter life, then you are not a real man – and you will never mature.

    You need to break out of the cycle – porn is not a pain reliever.

2. Do not make watching porn an option.
    Keep that mindset before you: it is not an option. The longer you go without porn, the longer it will not be an option. Think as if it doesn't exist at all then you will completely forget about it. When porn is non-existent in your mind, then you do not need to spend the day fighting your urge to watch it. You will not have to try so hard to avoid something that is non-existent. This way, you can dismiss your sexual urges right away.

3. Watch your urges mindfully.
    Do not react to your body's urges. You do not need to suppress or push them away them either. But observe carefully. And when you feel those urges hit, do something that can take your mind off the desire: take a walk, call a friend, meditate, exercise or take a cold shower – anything that will help you overcome. Pretty soon, you will not feel those urges again.

4. Do not focus on "not watching porn."
    Truth is, the more you think about avoiding something, the more you think about it. Keep it out of your mind and it will be soon out of your sight. The greater amount of though you give it, the less likely you can let it go. So just don't think about it, period.

5. Set realistic, achievable goals.
    Set smaller goals and certain milestones and work your way to one, little by little. When you get to one milestone, celebrate your mini-success and work in towards the next milestone. Do not be overambitious so that you

will not fall flat on your face and get discouraged when you don't meet goals. Learn to step back on previous successes to get strength to overcome the next hurdles.

6. Allow yourself to fail.
Give yourself room to grow, make mistakes, and get back up again. It is a process. Like riding a bike, no one can do it right away. You may need training wheels at first. Do not beat yourself up if you fall and don't quit. You will get better at it as you press on. One day, you will see that you can ride smoothly and not have trouble thinking about porn anymore.

7. Rebuild your lifestyle on a good foundation.

Addiction to porn can make one live out of control – lack of sleep, bad nutrition, no exercise, struggles in career, among others. The addict will treat himself so lowly because of the shame he feels. It is important to rebuild your lifestyle – get balance in every area of life. Learn to treat yourself as a beloved child. It is not selfish to enjoy life. Eat well, exercise, get a hobby. Have fun and enjoy life while you are recovering from your destructive behavior. Be positive!

8. Get this clear: watching porn is not a part of your life anymore.
Decide that porn is a thing of the past. Stop obsessing over your past. There is absolutely no need to blog about your struggle or hang on to recovery forums and mull about what you're going through. Focus on what is important now rather than what is behind. Set your mind on your dreams, your career, your family, your health. Then you will truly keep porn out of your system.

9. Get a support group.

Most people cannot accomplish anything extraordinary by themselves. You need other people to surround you with support and encouragement. Build a network with family, friends and a group who can help you stay on the road to recovery. Find people who you can deeply trust – people with whom you can share your struggles and small victories. They can help you through the confusion, discomfort and pain. When you feel that you are not alone in this journey, you can press on. Addiction can make you feel as the most awful and shameful person and will lead you to isolate yourself. To break this, travel with people with whom you can be honest and reveal your human, broken side.

Develop New Behaviors to Prevent Relapse

Contrary to what sex addicts think or feel, the truth is that no one gets real, long-term pleasure and satisfaction from sex addiction. All they get is a temporary and illusionary relief from the uncomfortable, nagging feelings brought about by their compulsive behavior.

Addiction is a process. One is not born a sex addict. In the early phase of his addiction, he sincerely believes that what he is doing causes him pleasure. When he is in the middle phase, he may question this pleasure, but continues with the behavior and the deeds. In the final phase, the sex addict realizes that he is creating for himself a world of pain instead of pleasure but doesn't stop his addiction. He is in a deep and destructive rut. People tend to label sex addicts who fail at making changes. They may call the addicts stupid, lazy, or self-destructive.

That is why it is important to use the right approach in overcoming an addiction. Otherwise, you will fail disastrously and further plunge yourself into the depths of your addiction. It is then that you will feel hopeless about change and settle for failures.

Here are some wrong ideas regarding treatments for sex addiction:

- People think that using medication is an answer. This is false because some drugs cause side effects that can be worse than sex addiction.
- People think that looking back into the past and analyzing a sex addict's childhood will help them. Some therapists waste time delving into what was but the problem is here and now – and that is what you should deal with.
- People think that behavior modification on the surface will eventually give the addict power over the addiction. Temporary solutions that do not address underlying addictive feelings will not help change a person.
- People think that repressing the sexual desires will control the addiction. Trying to stop the addiction by keeping the sexual desires inside will prove to be disastrous. When these desires surface, the sex addict will have no way to deal with it and will most likely have a relapse that is worse than his condition to begin with.
- People think that you can force a sex addict to stop. When you force sex addicts into stopping their compulsive acts, they may feel angry at at you for pressuring them into a new behavior. They may also feel depressed if they fail at a certain point, which will just worsen their behavior.

- People think that sex addiction is a disease and the addict is not responsible for his actions. A sex addict must realize that he IS responsible for the way he thinks and the things that he does.

In dealing with porn addiction and other sex addictions, there are significant risk factors that need acknowledgment and specific treatments. These include living a negligible life, giving up on real intimate sexual relationships, and falling into daily routines of sexual addiction practice such as porn use.

When these issues are not addressed, recovering sex addicts will find it difficult to recover from their addiction. They may even have frequent relapses because their behaviors have a powerful hold on them. Treatment and recovery may require following through with minimal planning for mindfulness strategies so that the behaviors can be controlled and stopped.

For example, getting rid of personal computers or simply using blocking software will prove to be an unreliable and temporary solution. It is only a form of repression. When a sex addict accidentally or unexpectedly encounters sexual imagery, he may fall into a relapse. Treatment should target the underlying issues of sex addiction.

Some sex addicts associate real intimacy with confusion and pain and they avoid reaching out and interacting with people. Most sex addicts, particularly those hooked with pornography, are isolated and emotionally insecure. To prevent relapse, an addict's behavior must be modified and he needs to develop new and healthy behaviors.

To accomplish this, he can do the following:

1. Vision: ap out a life that is full and bursting with exciting activities.

   A person who lives in isolation may be living in messy, unorganized surroundings. He has the tendency to be an under-earner or underachiever because of his emotional insecurity. To counter this life of deprivation, he must decide to make a long-term plan for a life of meaning and success.

   He must visualize himself as someone who is actually succeeding. This does not mean daydreaming or being in a fantasy. It means setting goals and doing everything possible to get those goals. It means being productive and not settling for unpaid activities. It may mean getting a better job and going with a new circle of friends. A recovering sex addict should make life goals his top priority. If he indulges in this objective as his main recovery activity, then he is less likely to suffer a relapse.

2. Change: Modify your daily routine or get out of an existing one.

The most dangerous behavior of sex addicts is the daily routine that they have. They get stuck in a rut that predictably gets them to end up in abnormal sexual activities. Being in an anti-social pothole can make one feel like a victim and give in to his compulsive behavior. However, if one changes his daily routine radically and does his best to put variety to it, then he will be able to set his mind on better things and more productive activities and eventually overcome his addiction without the risk of relapse.

3. Renew: Reclaim the concept of a good, intimate relationship.

The most important change that a sex addict can make is to change his mind about real, intimate, and healthy sexual relationships. Most sex addicts do not have a concept or have no good experience when it comes to intimacy. However, when they recover from their addiction, they can make new choices, practice new behaviors towards relationships, and become better at intimate relationships.

The biggest concern in treatment to recovery would be a sex addict's mindset. In his addiction, he has actually given up on the idea of being engaged in a real, intimate relationship. He might feel that it is impossible or too difficult. To address this, a sex addict must sensibly imagine what a good sexual relationship is. He must not fantasize about a perfect one but get a good, realistic concept of what a good sex life is.

It takes a lot to live life differently. On the road to recovery, you must be patient with yourself and yet very determined to make changes. It is crucial to catch yourself in weak moments to avoid lapsing into your old behaviors and patterns.

Overcoming sexual addiction necessitates mental health. In addition, the foundation for mental health is honesty. You will have to be honest enough to identify your addiction and communicate it to others who can help you. You need to be intentional about finding out the root cause of your compulsive behavior and sincerely try to make people aware. Honesty will open the door for you to bring change into your life.

If you are sexually addicted, you might excuse your behavior with thoughts that include "I am only relaxing" or "Everybody does it". And thoughts like these hinder you from identifying your problem. You will then have false ideas about relationships and think of sexual prowess as a manipulating tool over people. You may also be trapped into doing what you think others expect from you, believing that money or popularity will make you a better person or thinking that sex is the real and only meaning of a relationship.

Look at yourself closely and identify your core behavior problems. Changing towards having healthy mind starts with a healthy knowledge of yourself and allowing the people around you – family and friends – to know you better and understand you. All healthy personal and behavioral changes begin with an honest mind. When you are truthful with someone, you will not throw in lies and illusions. You will build trust and you will soon enjoy the lasting benefits of real, intimate relationships.

It is not a fairy tale: you really can overcome sex addiction. The length of your addiction does not matter. Recovery does not require wealth or popularity. You age, gender and cultural background is also not an issue.

Healthy Sexual Intimacy after Sex Addiction

It is a lie that you cannot enjoy the pleasures of real, intimate sex after recovering from sex addiction. On the contrary, you can still have a healthy sexual relationship. Even though sex addiction has given you perverted thoughts and inclinations about sex, it doesn't mean that you are stuck with that.

You can enjoy good, pleasurable sex with the one you love. First, you need to get a healthy mindset about sex so you will experience what healthy sexual relationships can bring.

1. Know that sex provides a general feeling of connection and well-being. In a healthy sexual relationship, people can feel safe, affirmed and connected. While it can take you time to get away from disconnection, shame and feelings of danger, you can get to the place where you are free to be yourself and enjoy sex. You just need some perseverance and patience.

2. Sex is not an outlet for your emotional expression. You can rediscover creative activities about closeness, such as intimate touches and playing soft music. In a healthy relationship, you do not need to be limited. You can revive passion and resourcefulness in sexual activities.

3. You realize that you can be vulnerable emotionally and it is acceptable. You do not have to fear betrayal or rejection. You do not need to sexualize your feelings to protect yourself. In healthy sexual relationships, you can be honest with yourself and your partner.

4. Healthy sexual intimacy will also give you the benefit of feeling physical and emotional sensations. You get to experience these feelings positively. When you are aware of your own physical sensations and your emotional vulnerability to the intimate relationship, you will find no need to focus on orgasm or to feel anesthetized. You will actually take pleasure in sex because you love the whole act.

5. A healthy mindset about sex can bring you to a level of self-nurture that is healthy and more authentic. You can experience pleasure deliberately and regularly without the shame and guilt.

6. You realize that you can cope up with suffering, disappointment, difficulties, and tiredness when you view them as a part of life. You do not have to turn to sexual relief to ease stress and tensions.

7. You can balance and moderate sexuality. Sexual maturity is about controlling an appropriate amount of sexual energy, not repressing it or expressing it excessively.

8. When you view sex as healthy, you develop healthy boundaries with other people. Sex addicts can be too rigid or too lax because they fail to recognize

the importance of boundaries to keep themselves and their partners safe. When you have and maintain healthy boundaries, you can be safe and vulnerable in your relationships.

9. Healthy sexual relationships allow you to trust other people. When you grow to trust yourself and recognize your truth, you also use the same healthy boundaries to trust others. In turn, you can progress in your relationships.

10. When you have a healthy mindset about sex, you become curious about people's responses to you and you become more caring. You refuse to take things personally, and you do not react emotionally. Healthy and mature intimacy gives you room to understand what's going on for you and for others during sex.

A Picture of Recovery from Sex Addiction

Sex addicts have led dysfunctional lives. During therapies and programs, they deal with their compulsive and dangerous behaviors. They take steps to change their behaviors and define mentalities that will help them understand beyond their addiction. Sometimes these strategies work out, at other times they don't. As a result, some relationships break down and others change for the better.

When sex addicts go to a rehabilitation program or therapy for their addiction, they are not sure how to recover. They think that there is no more life after sex addiction; this is a big lie.

If you are a sex addict on a recovery program, do not give up. There is hope: you can be a person that is better than the one you used to be. The key is you have to think of yourself as if you are an addict and not an adulterer. Help your spouse and the people you value to understand that you have an addiction so that they can help you get on the road to recovery and help you stay there.

This is a picture of what recovery can look like for you.

- You will have a real and more intimate relationship after building trust. Moreover, honesty will become the new foundation for this trust. You will enjoy sex more because of respect. Passion will grow when there are no more secrets.
- When you see a "trigger" you will not go back to it anymore. Cruising ignites the fuse, so they say. You do not repress your feelings, because you have the strength to say "no".
- You realize that sex addiction was not about sex after all. It only looks like sex, but is actually a void in your life that you are trying to fill. With addiction, you avoid real intimacy with people you love because you replace them with connections from strangers and wanton sexual activities. It may have taken you time to realize that all this was nonsense but righting all the wrongs will be very profitable for you and your spouse/partner.
- You do not flirt anymore – you realize that flirting is never innocent. If there are instances that you may do so, you immediately let your spouse or partner know. Openness gives you the strength to overcome. You know that your spouse will eventually find out anyway and it is best to be honest now. The more your practice honesty, the more it becomes ingrained in your life. The easier your days ahead will become.

The road to stopping the compulsive behavior is demanding and quite complex. Honesty makes it harder to travel that road – but it is the only way to be free. If you will look at addiction and call it as it is, then you will not make excuses for your behavior. You will not find reasons to get off the road. You will not call bad behavior as innocent.

Accountability is also crucial. When you have recovered from addiction, you will have the joy to experience new relationships or enhance your existing ones. To keep you on track, you may need accountability tools. You have to know that addictions are very crafty devils. They can set you up and jump on you without you knowing it.

An example of accountability tool is the polygraph test. It will help you uncover everything. It will also make you take stock of what you have done in the previous year or month that can be slips in your behavior. It is important to identify these slips so they do not remain unchecked. Some people fail these tests for the simple reason that they have something to hide. Your goal is not to simply pass the test, but to maintain a life that is free from lies. You undergo this test to make sure that lying will not be an option for you. It is like confirming that you are living up to your end of the bargain to change.

Recovery is different for everybody. Some people just drop all the activities altogether. Some can still enjoy doing the things they used to do before – only this time, they do it with their wife and only when it feels right to do so. For example, a person who has recovered from sex addiction can have an active, intimate relationship with his wife and go with her to strip clubs on occasion. The reason behind it is that they have agreed that they can share the fun, sexy experience of the club together.

However, the good picture is this: the former sex addict does not do it by himself; he does not go on shameful nights of sexual adventures. He can go to strip clubs with his wife because there are no secrets. He can even masturbate in her presence when it is comfortable for both of them. He does not do it when he is alone because he protects the intimate, sexual connection he has with his wife. There is no more fantasy world for him, only a real intimate relationship.

You have to realize that sex is a good thing; it is for pleasure, not perversion. People who love each other should just explore sex and not abuse each other. Sex is not about losing dignity and respect, but gaining an appreciation of who you are in the course of intimacy.

Recovery from sex addiction looks like this: a life without secrets. It is the end of the end of dangerous and compulsive sexual behaviors. While there are still challenges and temptations in your way, you can have the strength to overcome them and live a full and happy life.

Bonus Chapter: Recovery for Partners of Sex Addicts

Sex addiction is a real problem that causes real destruction to relationships. The emotional involvement of people who are in a complex relationship with sex addicts can be very challenging. They will most likely experience emotional peaks and valleys as they are affected by betrayals. Even as the sex addict will go through stages in his recovery, the partner will also have his or her own journey.

Following are six identifiable phases of recovery for people who are involved with sex addicts, particularly spouses/partners:

1. Early development (An initial realization of the problem)
2. Crisis (Information gathering and Decision)
3. Shock (Highly emotional stage of confusion and aversion)
4. Grief or Ambivalence (Acceptance and inward focus)
5. Repair (Self-Nurture)
6. Growth (Maturity)

The first phase of recovery is the early development stage. This is the period before the partner gets to discover the reality of the addict's problem. The partner has no knowledge of the addict's compulsive behavior. He or she does not have suspicions that there is something wrong with their relationship. However, he or she may feel difficulty in some areas of their relationship: intimacy, parenting, finances, etc. When addressing these issues, the sex addict will deny that there is a problem. However, the partner should persist in finding out the cause for concern to get to the next phase eventually.

In the next phase, the partner discovers the sexual compulsive behavior of the sex addict. In the beginning, the partner will have the tendency to adopt various techniques and strategies to help the addict. One reason why a partner may try everything to help the addict is he or she does not want to feel the betrayal and rejection. At the crisis phase, the partner begins gathering information and resources to get the addict on the road to change and recovery. It can be by reading books, through counseling with a sex addiction therapist or by attending 12-step groups.

The following stage is the phase of shock. It can be a serious and highly emotional phase involving avoidance, numbness, and periods of conflict between the partner and the sex addict. It is a normal phase to go through but it is very painful because violent feelings may arise such as hopelessness, resentment, self-doubt and anger. Both the sex addict and his or her partner will need enough emotional and mental support to get him or her through this difficult period.

After shock comes self-doubt and grief. The partner will eventually feel the weight of the emotional upheaval and may focus inward to grieve about his or her loss. It is the time to when the partner focuses less on the sex addict's behavior and compulsiveness. It is the time to look beyond the feelings of betrayal. It is the time to when the partner looks within and starts taking care of himself physically, mentally and emotionally – to get beyond his or her own uncertainty.

The next phase after grieving is repair. The partner should be, at this time, entirely focused on investing in self-care. After the grieving process, he or she should develop an emotional stability through healthy boundaries. The partner can get out of the relationship or decide to stay – whether or not the sex addict is on a strong and solid recovery program. If they decide to stick it out, they should however, set defined guidelines and healthy boundaries that will protect both of them as they build on a new level of relationship.

The last phase of recovery is growth or maturity. Initially, the partner may have felt victimized. Nevertheless, he can bounce back and have a healthy, strong, and successful intimate relationship again. There will be a solid commitment to maturity and healing through acceptance and adjustments from both parties.

Just as a sex addict's recovery program can take months or years, the same goes for his or her partner. It will take time, depending on various factors, for the partner to get through recovery. Partners can take advantage of professional treatments, support groups, and various resources. Just like sex addicts, they need all the help they can get. The good news is that they can go through this and it should not be a roadblock for growth. They can enjoy life, intimacy, and healthy sex after being partners with victims of sex addiction.

Conclusion

Thank you again for downloading this book!

I hope this book has given you ample information about sex addiction and how to overcome it. Overcoming sex addiction is not easy but it can be done. If you set your mind to it, you can be successful. It can be a long process, but it will surely bring you a new sense of life and love. All the times that you missed out on the fulfillment that intimacy brings can be restored.

The next step is to put to use all the information you have learned. Recognize your need for help to make room for change and growth. There is so much more to life than your addiction. You are stronger than you think! You can conquer this weakness and enjoy physical, emotional and relational stability.

Get on the road to recovery – you can do it!

Finally, if you enjoyed this book, it will be greatly appreciated if you can please take the time to share your thoughts and post a review on Amazon.

Thank you and good luck!

One Last Thing...

If you enjoyed this book or found it useful I'd be very grateful if you'd post a short review on Amazon. Your support really does make a difference and I read all the reviews personally so I can get your feedback and make this book even better.

If you'd like to leave a review then all you need to do is click the review link on this book's page...

Thank You so Much

www.ingramcontent.com/pod-product-compliance
Lightning Source LLC
Chambersburg PA
CBHW071346310526
45790CB00018B/1371